Stuttering

The Disorder of Many Theories

GERALD JONAS

Routledge & Kegan Paul

London and Henley

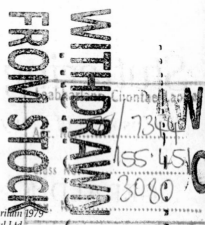

First published in Great Britain 1979
by Routledge & Kegan Paul Ltd
39 Store Street, London WC1E 7DD and
Broadway House, Newtown Road,
Henley-on-Thames, Oxon RG9 1EN
Printed in Great Britain by
Redwood Burn Ltd, Trowbridge and Esher

British Library Cataloguing in Publication Data

Jonas, Gerald

Stuttering

1: Stuttering
I. Title
616.8' 554   RC 424   79-40200

ISBN 0 7100 0286 6
ISBN 0 7100 0287 4 Pbk

To my mother & father

Stuttering

The Disorder of Many Theories

WHAT I REMEMBER MOST acutely about my stuttering is not the strangled sound of my own voice but the impatient looks on other people's faces when I had trouble getting a word out. And if their eyes happened to reflect some of the pain and frustration I was feeling, that only made me more uneasy. There was nothing they could do to help me, and I certainly didn't want their sympathy. I was nine or ten at the time. Like most people with a stuttering problem, I had already learned to live by my wits in a way that normally fluent people cannot begin to appreciate. Whenever I opened my mouth, I mentally glanced ahead at the

3

sentence I wanted to say, to see if there was any word I was likely to stutter on. For me, speaking was like riding down a highway and reading aloud from a series of billboards. I knew that to speak normally I had to keep moving forward at a steady pace. Yet every once in a while I became aware of an obstacle, like an enormous boulder, blocking the road some five or six billboards ahead of me. I knew that when I got to that particular word I would be unable to say it. I never figured out why I stuttered on one word rather than another. Some sounds—like the "m" sound at the beginning of a word—were particularly troublesome; but, even with these, the context was all-important. A sentence might have two words beginning with "m," such as "I'll have to ask my mother." The moment I framed this sentence in my mind, I knew that I would have no trouble pronouncing "my" but that "mother" would be impossible. My usual strategy at such times was to speed up and try to crash through the obstacle. When I succeeded, the sentence came out like this: "I'll [pause for deep breath] havetoaskmymother." This trick worked just often enough to convince some people that I stuttered because I talked too fast. But when it failed I found myself struck dumb in midsentence, unable to go forward or turn back.

4

There were times when I got as far as the first sound in the difficult word and could do nothing but repeat it like a broken record, in the classic stutter that is imitated—usually for laughs—in books and movies. More often, I had a complete block; I would try to form the first sound in the word and something inside me would snap shut, so that if I opened my mouth nothing came out.

At that point, I usually backed up and looked for a detour. Sometimes all I had to do was find a less troublesome word that meant the same thing. For example, I might be able to get away with something like "I'll have to check with my folks." If I couldn't think of a synonym quickly enough, I had no choice but to rephrase the sentence, to try to sneak up on the difficult word from another direction; the result might come out as: "You know how mothers are, I better ask her first." I didn't have the slightest idea why the same word should be easier to say in one context than in another, but whenever it worked out that way I felt an absurd pride in my accomplishment; no one else knew that in order to speak with any fluency I had to become a kind of walking thesaurus. But the strategies of substitution and circumlocution created their own problems. The further I strayed from the original wording of the sentence, the more I had to guard against letting subtle changes of meaning creep in. If I wasn't careful, I could find myself saying things I didn't quite mean, just to be able to say something. In a way, my situation was not so different from that of a writer in a totalitarian country who tries to communicate under the constant threat of censorship. The fact that I carried the censor around inside my head did not make the situation any less oppressive.

I don't remember exactly when I stopped stuttering. I seem to have outgrown the problem sometime during my adolescence. By the time I graduated from college, it had faded into a childhood nightmare—except for two mercifully brief relapses in my early twenties. In both cases, I found myself in social situations where I desperately wanted to be charming and witty and persuasive, and in both cases I got drunk and ended up completely blocked, unable to make a sound, let alone pronounce a word. In both cases, I was back to normal the next morning.

I still talk too fast, according to my parents (and now my parents-in-law); and occasionally I stumble over a word or two when I'm nervous, as many people do. But speech holds no special terrors for me. Indeed, the more nervous I get, the more I talk. People who did not know me as a child are surprised when I tell them I once had a stuttering problem. Looking back, I can hardly believe it myself. Anyone who has met an adult chronic stutterer knows how terrible an affliction stuttering can be. The classic symptoms of stuttering (or "stammering," an older usage, which is still preferred in England) include rapid-fire repetitions of consonant or vowel sounds, especially at the beginning of words; unnaturally prolonged vowel sounds in the middle of words; and complete verbal blocks. The last, of course, are the worst. In the struggle to terminate a block, some stutterers become so agitated that they resemble an epileptic having an attack: cold sweat appears on their foreheads, they gasp for breath, their eyes bulge, their lips quiver, their arms jerk like a puppet's, they spray saliva in all directions; they seem to be literally trying to shake the words loose from their tongue. It is not hard to see why such people were once thought to be possessed by demons; when chronic stutterers talk about themselves, they often refer to their body as if it were under alien control. "My lips refuse to open," they say, or, "My tongue gets stuck to my jaw."

The chronic stutterer knows that he is not suffering from any ordinary speech impediment, like a lisp or slurred vowels caused by bad bite. The ability to communicate through language defines us as human beings in a human society. When men learned to speak, they set themselves off from all other creatures. Stuttering strikes at the very root of this distinction. Most of us have stuttered at times when we were in a hurry or anxious or frightened. But only a few people become chronic stutterers. When I was growing up, I was often told that I stuttered because my mind worked faster than my mouth. (Or was it the other way around?) I was also assured that if a natural left-hander was forced to do things right-handed, he would end up stuttering; and the same was supposedly true of people who got a terrible scare at a young age. I never believed that any of these explanations applied to me. They sounded too much like old wives' tales—on the order of the stories that attributed little Johnny's musical talent to all the records his mother listened to during her last weeks of pregnancy.

Not long ago, I decided to satisfy my curiosity by looking into the voluminous scientific literature that has grown up around stuttering. I had no trouble finding explanations of why people start to stutter. Indeed, I found a grab bag of competing and often contradictory explanations—some of which bore a suspicious resemblance to the old wives' tales I remembered from my childhood. But the first, and possibly the most significant, thing I learned was that nothing about stuttering is as simple as it seems—for the reason that nothing about speech is as simple as it seems.

Stuttering has been called "the disorder of many theories." Over the years, the symptoms of stuttering have been attributed to a number of causes, including a broad range of organic defects, neuroses of one kind or another, social pressures, faulty learning experiences, and endless combinations of these factors. The conflicts of opinion among the experts are hardly academic, since each theory implies a different kind of therapy, and many of the leading authorities on stuttering during the last half century have themselves been life-long stutterers. I cannot think of another branch of science or medicine in which the biblical adjuration "Physician, heal thyself" is so poignantly applicable. It is true that all psychoanalysts go through some form of psychotherapy during training, but they rarely write about their own neuroses in the psychoanalytic journals. In the literature on stuttering, however, the dry prose of the objective scientist will suddenly give way to passages of almost confessional intensity—

especially when the author is explaining why the long-sought cure for stuttering remains out of reach.

There are certain hard facts about stuttering that everyone agrees *ought* to provide some clues to its underlying nature. Unfortunately, the clues seem to point in several directions at once. Innumerable surveys have established that in Western countries, no matter what language or local dialect is spoken, about 1 percent of the population has a stuttering problem. (The United States is estimated to have two million stutterers today.) The same surveys show that young males are much more likely than young females to become stutterers—by a ratio of three or four to one, according to some researchers. Twins of both sexes seem to stutter more than other people. Among identical twins (who develop from a single fertilized egg), if one twin stutters, the other twin almost invariably does too. Among fraternal twins (who develop from two eggs and so do not share the same genetic makeup), there is a much better chance that one twin will stutter while the other will not.

One way to account for all these figures is to assume that people stutter because of a genetically transmitted flaw—a defect in the speech apparatus or a "miswired" circuit in the nervous system—

that reliably shows up in a certain subgroup of the population, like birthmarks or color blindness or male-pattern baldness. So far, however, all attempts to identify the physiological basis of stuttering have failed. In fact, investigators have failed to detect any obvious difference between people who stutter and people who don't. This may not be surprising in light of another finding: the problem of stuttering typically appears between the ages of three and five, *after* the child has already made great strides toward fluency. In other words, the mechanism works well enough when it is first set in motion; the trouble comes later, just as speech is becoming less of a feat and more of a habit.

Some observers argue that since stuttering has not been shown to have a physiological basis, it must be a neurotic symptom whose origin should be sought in the unresolved conflicts of early childhood. Just as certain people express their neuroses through sick headaches, and others by eating too much, the stutterer may have deep-seated personality problems that find expression—or, rather, nonexpression—in speech blocks and repetitions. The one thing that virtually every stutterer has trouble with is his own name—particularly when he is called upon to identify himself to someone in authority. But if stuttering is a neurotic symptom, why do countless objective studies using standard diagnostic tests indicate that stutterers are no more neurotic than the rest of the population? And why have so many psychotherapists (starting with Freud himself) conceded that their methods are not much help in straightening out the speech of patients who stutter? No one doubts that chronic stutterers have personality problems. The question is, which comes first—the stuttering or the problems? It would take a strong personality indeed to remain unmarked by the experience of picking up a telephone and staring into the mouthpiece, unable to speak, while the person on the other end says, with mounting annoyance, "Hello? Hello? Who is this? Is anybody there?"

There is one fact about stuttering so obvious that its significance is often overlooked: no one stutters all the time. Most chronic stutterers have certain words that almost always give them trouble in ordinary conversation; these are known as Jonah words, for obvious reasons. But the same words—or the same sounds, at least—will flow effortlessly from the stutterer's lips if he is conversing in a foreign language, or talking in a funny accent, or singing, or reciting a sentence in unison with someone else. Even the most severely handicapped stutterer—the young man, say, who goes through fearsome contortions to get out a few words to a girl at a party—will be able to articulate with ease when he is talking to a small child, or to a dog or some other animal, or to his own reflection in the bathroom mirror.

Since the pressure to communicate can make stuttering worse, it has been suggested that social pressure is to blame for stuttering in the first place. According to one theory, a child starts to stutter because he is overaware of the need to use the "correct" word, the "correct" accent, and so on. Proponents of this theory cite the curious fact that several American Indian tribes in the Midwest—among them the Utes and the Bannocks—have virtually no stuttering problem. It happens that these tribes also have a remarkably permissive attitude toward children's speech. By contrast, their distant cousins in the Pacific Northwest, the Cowichans, expect children to take part at an early age in complicated rituals under the critical eyes and ears of the tribal elders. The Cowichans, who place a premium on verbal skills, have a highly competitive society—and a high incidence of stuttering.

It may well be that the reason the children of the

Utes and the Bannocks do not stutter is that no one ever tries to make them speak "correctly." But the theory fails to explain why in so many other cultures some children of nagging parents turn into stutterers while others do not. In trying to account for the known facts about stuttering without playing down individual and cultural differences, some researchers have emphasized that stuttering is essentially learned behavior—a speech habit ingrained in a child as a result of certain childhood experiences and periodically reinforced during normal social intercourse. Taking their cues from Ivan Pavlov and B. F. Skinner, a number of behavioral therapists have recently attempted to cure stuttering by breaking the old patterns of reinforcement. Their preliminary reports of success must be evaluated with great care, for stuttering is notoriously susceptible to the so-called placebo effect. The most severe case will respond temporarily to almost any form of therapy, no matter how bizarre, as long as the stutterer thinks he is in good hands. Furthermore, recent studies have shown that as many as four fifths of all young children who are labeled stutterers simply stop stuttering by the end of adolescence—as I did—without any treatment whatever.

For all these reasons, stuttering therapy has

always been a fruitful field for faith healers of various persuasions, for overenthusiastic amateurs, and for outright charlatans. Since even the adult severe stutterer can speak fluently some of the time, a "cure" always seems tantalizingly close. And the same scenario has been repeated time and time again in history: high hopes prematurely aroused, only to be cruelly disappointed.

A heartfelt prayer to be relieved of the anguish of stuttering has been found on a cuneiform tablet from Mesopotamia, dated several centuries before Christ. There is no indication that the prayer was answered. When the voice from the burning bush commanded Moses to lead his people out of Egypt, Moses protested that he was "slow of speech, and of a slow tongue," and legend has it that his problem was a stutter. We know on the authority of the Old Testament that the problem was solved not by a miracle but by an evasion. When the time came to inform the Israelites of God's command, it was his brother Aaron who "spake all the words which the Lord had spoken unto Moses." What may be the first recorded cure for stuttering is described in a Greek myth about a young prince named Battus, who beseeched the oracle at Delphi to unscramble his speech. In its usual roundabout way, the oracle told Battus to gather an army, sail to North Africa, subdue the hostile inhabitants, and never return. Despite his stuttered reply that he was not the man for the job, Battus obeyed, and, the tale concludes, he not only triumphed in battle but spoke happily ever after as the golden-tongued ruler of the Greek colony of Cyrene.

The implied moral—that a stutterer can be cured by a drastic change of environment—gives the myth of Battus a strangely modern ring. (Behavior therapy says much the same thing, in a different jargon.) The most famous of all myths about stuttering—the story of Demosthenes, who learned to speak clearly by outshouting the surf through a mouthful of pebbles—suggests that stuttering is a problem of misarticulation which can be overcome with practice. Whatever the value of these mythological insights, the more down-to-earth Greeks were convinced that stuttering was caused by some gross physical defect of the speech organs, and this insight dominated Western medical thought for the next two millennia.

Aristotle, who some authorities say stuttered himself, believed that the stutterer's tongue was abnormally thick or hard, and so was "too sluggish to keep pace with the imagination." Hippocrates put the blame on an excessively dry tongue, and he prescribed blistering substances to drain away the "black bile" causing the trouble. The Roman physician Celsus suggested gargling and massages to strengthen a weak tongue. And Galen, the second-century Greek physician, who was looked upon as the supreme medical authority in Europe during the Middle Ages, thought that the stutterer's tongue was too cold and wet. In the early seventeenth century, Francis Bacon approached the problem with a mind trained in the new scientific empiricism; he concluded that many people stuttered because of "the Refrigeration of the tongue, whereby it is less apt to move." To thaw the stiff tongue he suggested a draught of hot wine.

The long tradition of "curing" a stutterer by correcting some imagined defect of the tongue reached a horrifying climax in the first half of the nineteenth century, when the Prussian surgeon Johann Friedrich Dieffenbach decided that people stuttered because their tongues were too large. Fitting practice to theory in a number of cases, Dieffenbach proceeded to cut the excessive organs down to size by snipping off chunks from the sides. According to his own testimony, these operations were highly successful.

Partly in reaction to such abuses, other investigators in the early nineteenth century began to explore the possibility that stuttering was caused by some kind of "nervous condition" or "predisposition." But since the nervous system itself was then largely beyond the reach of medical science, therapeutic attention was focused on the stutterer's outward symptoms, especially abnormal breathing and faulty coordination of the speech organs. The nineteenth century was, after all, the heyday of elocution. The mastery of public speaking was considered an important accomplishment for the educated classes (and a virtual necessity for the socially ambitious parvenu). The basic premise of the elocutionary movement was that most people picked up bad speech habits during childhood, and that these habits could be eradicated if the individual was taught the "proper" use of his speech organs. With this as a working hypothesis, many professors of elocution took it upon themselves to treat the symptoms of stuttering without worrying much about the underlying causes.

In 1841, Professor Andrew Comstock, of the Vocal and Polyglott Gymnasium in Philadelphia, laid out a detailed therapeutic program for stuttering which began with breathing exercises and built up through the diligent practice of individual sounds, words, and phrases, until the student was ready to "commit to memory a short piece which requires to be spoken with explosive force; for example 'Satan's Speech to his Legions' " (from Milton's *Paradise Lost*). Soon after, in England, Alexander Melville Bell, a famous teacher of the deaf (whose son later invented the telephone), made an even stronger case for the elocutionary approach to the treatment of "stammering." In *The Principles of Speech and Vocal Physiology*, he decried the "professional dogma and popular delusion" that a stammer was caused by some kind of organic defect. It was nothing but a bad habit, Bell insisted, and you cannot "excise a habit" with a scalpel or dose it with a tonic. Instead of seeking help from surgeons and physicians, Bell said, the person who stammered should spend his time "reeducating" his unruly speech organs: "Let the stammerer particularly attend to the disposition of his lips . . . to prevent their officious meddling with sounds over which they have no legitimate influence." To keep the teeth in line, Bell suggested speaking aloud while biting down firmly on the blade of a paper cutter. The tongue, which Bell characterized as "the most alert and obedient organ in the body," should not give too much trouble: "This member is fairly easily disciplined to good habits and broken off from bad ones."

Another theory that was very much in vogue in the nineteenth century was that stuttering could be "contagious"—in the sense that one child would begin to stutter in conscious imitation of another child and soon find himself unable to stop. The suggested remedy: weed all stutterers out of your child's circle of playmates.

Of all the early attempts to explain stuttering as a perverse misuse of fundamentally healthy organs, my favorite is a little book entitled *Shut Your Mouth*, by George Catlin, the American portrait painter who achieved fame as a frontier artist. During his lengthy travels with various tribes of Plains Indians, Catlin made two shrewd observations: unlike the slack-jawed white settlers, the Indians kept their lips firmly sealed most of the time; and when they did open their mouths to speak, they never stuttered. Putting one and one together, Catlin concluded that stuttering was caused by "a nervous hesitation and vibration of the underjaw when brought up from its habitual hanging state to perform its part in articulation." A comparison of "savage and civilized human beings" revealed "the necessity and desirability to keep the mouth closed, except during speaking and taking food." Snoring was also to be avoided.

There are no statistics to tell us whether more stutterers were helped by the methods of Comstock and Bell than by the advice of Catlin. At least, Bell was a serious student of speech problems who promised no easy cures. But the elocutionary approach lent itself all too readily to exploitation, in the form of commercial stuttering schools operated by people with little training and few scruples. Before agreeing to perform a "cure" for a fat fee, these practitioners would swear the stutterers to eternal silence about the methods to be used. In most cases, the treatment was based on the well-known fact that stutterers temporarily stop stuttering when they are distracted from their usual speech patterns. Since almost any novel stimulus will serve as a distraction (until the novelty wears off), the stuttering schools taught their students to rely on such gimmicks as talking with a singsong inflection, talking with an exaggerated drawl, and talking while tapping a finger, swinging the arms, or stamping a foot.

In between practice sessions, the students were given pep talks to build up their confidence and strengthen their "will." At the same time, they were told to forgo all attempts at ordinary conversation until the end of the treatment—which might take weeks, or even months. Once a stutterer had learned to speak fluently within the confines of the school, he was considered ready to resume his normal life. The practitioner had little to fear from an unsatisfied customer. When the inevitable relapse occurred—when the distracting gimmicks no longer distracted and the artificially bolstered self-confidence faltered—the abject stutterer would be the last person in the world to demand his money back.

Despite the legions of quacks and charlatans that the elocutionary movement harbored, it did provide the germ of the science of speech pathology. Bell once compared the job of a speech instructor to that of a music teacher giving flute lessons. Obviously, the first qualification for such a job is a thorough understanding of the instrument. And if the elocutionists' efforts to teach fluent speech to stutterers proved anything, it was that no one knew very much about the speech instrument.

The sounds of human speech are normally produced by "playing" on the outgoing stream of air as we exhale. Once the air leaves the chest cavity, it flows past a series of muscular baffles and valves that partly or completely impede its passage for varying lengths of time. In the larynx, or voice box, the moving air sets into vibration two small folds of flesh known as the vocal cords. These serve as the reeds of the speech instrument. By altering the tension and configuration of the vocal cords, the speaker can alter the pitch of the sounds that issue from his throat. These laryngeal sounds are in large part the raw material of speech. Shaping this material into the infinitely varied vowels and consonants of all the languages on earth requires exquisitely modulated changes in the tension, position, and configuration of the lips, tongue, jaws, cheeks, velum (or soft palate), and other structures in the so-called vocal cavity. As many as seventy-five muscles may be called into play during the production of a simple "mama." And, of course, each movement must come in exactly on cue. It does no good to set the lips for an "m" sound if you are inhaling, or to purse your lips for a "u" sound if your glottis has just closed and shut off the flow of air from the windpipe. Such attempts to defy the laws of physics have actually been observed during severe stuttering blocks.

By the beginning of the twentieth century, enough was known about the physiology of speech to convince even the most enthusiastic elocutionist that stuttering was no simple speech impediment, traceable to a physical defect like a misshapen palate or buckteeth. Certainly, there was something wrong with a person who repeatedly tried to make an "m" sound while inhaling; but the trouble seemed to be in his head, not in his mouth or throat. Some researchers took this insight quite literally; for them, stuttering was a symptom of a damaged or defective brain. This view was popular in Germany, where a school of speech pathologists tried to trace the difficulty to one cerebral structure or another.

Other investigators, who adopted the vocabulary and methods of Sigmund Freud, began searching for the cause—and cure—of stuttering in the regions of the unconscious. Freud himself had failed to relieve one of his early patients of a bad stutter; and he expressed doubt that psychoanalysis was an appropriate way to treat this complaint. But his followers were less cautious. Everyone agreed that stuttering was a neurotic symptom; the dispute began over what neurosis it was a symptom of. One analyst argued that stutterers were fixated at the infantile stage of "oral eroticism." Did not the compulsive repetition of lip and tongue movements represent "an act of nursing at an imaginary nipple"? Another analyst located the fixation at a different level: "One may speak, in stuttering, of a displacement upward of the functions of the anal sphincters." A German researcher identified a specific kind of stutter—*Spuckstottern*, in which the stutterer sprays the listener with saliva—as a sign of barely veiled aggression. (According to this interpretation, the stutterer is really saying "On the whole, I am glad that I can spit at you.") Stuttering was also seen as expressing a general ambivalence about communication: the person stutters because he desperately wants to talk to someone but is afraid of revealing what he considers to be his literally unspeakable desires and fantasies.

No matter what else they argued about, the psychoanalysts and the psychiatrists were all convinced of one thing: that it would be futile to try to cure a person's stutter without treating his underlying personality problems. Even if the stutter could be cleared up by purely symptomatic therapy, the neurotic would need something else to blame all his shortcomings on—and in due time another, possibly less attractive symptom would appear in place of the speech impediment.

Just when the psychoanalytical approach seemed most strongly entrenched in the United States, a new theory, based on the latest neurological insights, pointed toward a very subtle kind of organic defect as the cause of stuttering. Almost all the muscles involved in speech—from those that control the vocal cords to those that move the jaw up and down—are arranged in bilateral pairs. To produce intelligible speech, the muscles on one side of the body must move in perfect synchrony with the muscles on the other side. For instance, when I want to say "pop," both sides of my mouth must open and close at the same time; even a slight discrepancy in timing will garble the sound. In the fine tuning of the vocal cords, the margin for error is even smaller.

Because of the way the nervous system is organized, the muscles on the left side of the body are controlled by signals from the right hemisphere of the brain, and vice versa. Obviously, neither hemisphere can act in total isolation from the other, or there would be chaos instead of finely coordinated movement. What is not so obvious is how the coordination is achieved. By the late nineteen-twenties, there was good reason to believe that the left hemisphere of the brain is normally dominant; that is, it sets the pace and imposes its pattern of timing on the right hemisphere for many bilateral functions, including speech. The best evidence for this "cerebral dominance" came from case histories of brain-damaged patients; tumors or lesions on the left side of the brain were much more likely to produce serious speech deficits than identical damage on the right side. Of course, if the left cerebral hemisphere was normally dominant, this would also explain why most people are right-handed. In left-handed people, presumably, the right hemisphere played the dominant role. The trouble with stutterers—according to a theory advanced in 1927 by Lee Travis, the director of the University of Iowa Speech Clinic, and Dr. Samuel Orton, the chairman of the university's department of psychiatry—was that neither hemisphere was dominant enough. Instead of one side of the brain acting as a tyrant to oversee all muscular activity, the two hemispheres competed for control of every movement. To explain how this state of cerebral anarchy might come about, Orton and Travis speculated that many stutterers had been born left-handed but had been forced to do things with their right hands as children. This had "strengthened" the left side of the brain at the expense of the right—not enough to reverse the dominance but enough to prevent either side from exercising firm control. The resulting lack of synchrony might not be so evident in large-scale motor functions—like walking—but it could be disastrous for a person trying to speak.

One possible cure immediately suggested itself:

take all right-handed stutterers and switch them back to being lefties. To test this hypothesis, Orton and Travis needed a human guinea pig— someone with a severe stutter who was willing to undertake the difficult task of reeducating his neuromuscular-control system. They found the ideal candidate in a young Kansan named Wendell Johnson, who had come to the University of Iowa in the fall of 1926 because of its reputation as a leading research center for stuttering. He was twenty years old, and he had been stuttering since the age of six. His stutter was so severe that when he met Travis for the first time and handed him a letter of introduction, he was unable to utter so much as a "hello."

A few years earlier, Johnson had attended a commercial stuttering school, where he spent three months learning to speak in a "drawling monotone," and swinging dumbbells while chanting in a loud voice such inspirational slogans as "Have more backbone and less wishbone" and "Little drops of water wear away a rock." The stuttering school had been an expensive and humiliating failure. But that did not dim his enthusiasm for Travis's proposal, which was based, after all, not on quackery but on science.

Although Johnson had been doing most things

right-handed for as long as he could remember—and doing them well enough to be acclaimed as a schoolboy athlete in his home town—he accepted the suggestion that he had begun using his right hand only in unconscious imitation of other members of his family. And he set out to become a "thoroughgoing left-handed person" in the hope that this would, as he put it, "reestablish my native dominance in its original intensity." During the first few years of the experiment, he kept a written record of his thoughts and feelings, which was published in book form in 1930 under the title *Because I Stutter*. At this time, Johnson was convinced that he had finally found the source of his trouble. "The severity of my stuttering has declined markedly, and my attitude toward stuttering has changed enormously," he wrote. "I have stripped from my speech defect its ominous mystery." Alas, his optimism was premature. In another book, *Stuttering and What You Can Do About It*, published in 1961, he looked back at the results of all his hard work: "Ten years and countless bruises later, having become a threat to my own thumbs, I placed in storage [my] many ingenious braces and mittens . . . put away my left-handed scissors, and with my right hand wrote 'Finis' to the experiment, still stuttering splendidly."

By 1940, Johnson was on his way to becoming *the* authority on stuttering in the United States. As Travis's associate and eventually his successor at the Iowa Speech Clinic, Johnson began to focus his attention on the social context in which stuttering develops. Johnson's theory about the cause of stuttering, which has been called the "diagnosogenic" or "semantogenic" theory, grew out of a simple but startling observation: Stuttering is a social disease in the truest sense—you get it only because someone else says you have it. Johnson declared that the stutterer's trouble began *not* with a faulty nervous system but with a faulty diagnosis, usually by his parents. Every young child occasionally hesitates in his speech, repeats syllables, gropes for words, and in general has difficulty saying what is on his mind. According to a study conducted by one of Johnson's graduate students, these normal childhood "disfluencies" occur on the average of fifty times for every thousand words spoken. For instance, a child may come running into the house shouting, "I-I-I-I want some ice cream." Most parents will ignore the rapid repetition; they may not even be aware of it, because they are concentrating on what the child is saying and not on how he is saying it. Some adults, however, will do just the opposite.

They worry about the way their child speaks. They assume that he should be able to speak perfectly by the age of three or four, and when he fails to live up to their expectations, they begin to think of him as a stutterer. Inevitably, the child senses their concern—and the effect on his speech is disastrous, Johnson says. The child "learns to doubt that he can talk smoothly enough to please the people he talks to, mainly his parents," and, "He learns to fear what will happen if he doesn't. What this amounts to is that he learns to be afraid that 'he will stutter.' Naturally, therefore, he tries to do anything and everything he can think of to 'keep from stuttering.' Instead of just talking, he tries to talk 'without stuttering,' by doing things like pressing his lips together tightly, or holding his breath—but these are the things he does that he, and everyone else, calls his stuttering. Stuttering then is what the stutterer does trying not to stutter." Confused and embarrassed by his apparent failure to control his speech apparatus, the child eventually accepts the notion that there is something deeply wrong with him. And once he has labeled himself a "stutterer" his chances of escaping the vicious circle are slim indeed.

Johnson's theory was based not on his own childhood memories—he could not recall his parents making any fuss about his speech before he was six—but on hundreds of interviews with parents of stutterers who had brought their children to the Iowa Speech Clinic for treatment. The attitudes of these parents were compared with the attitudes of a control group whose children did not stutter. Johnson found that the parents of most stutterers tended to be perfectionists in their own lives; they were also upwardly mobile, in the sense that they wanted their children to do much better economically and socially than they had done, and they took it for granted that their children's success would depend to a great extent on how well they spoke. This assessment of the social arena may very well have been accurate, as George Bernard Shaw's Professor Higgins demonstrated in *Pygmalion*. But, unlike Professor Higgins, who knew exactly what Eliza Doolittle was capable of, the parents Johnson interviewed apparently made demands on their children that the average child simply could not meet. As Johnson saw it, the preponderance of male stutterers around the world simply proved that parents are generally more concerned about the way their male children speak.

Up to this point in my research, I had managed to maintain a fairly detached, "objective" attitude toward the material. One did not have to be an ex-stutterer to wince at the thought of Hippocrates' patients having their tongues blistered, or to shudder at Dieffenbach's criminal use of the scalpel, or to sympathize with the endless parade of stutterers who wasted their time and money seeking a miracle cure. But reading Johnson was different. When he described how stuttering developed in childhood, I began to get the uncomfortable feeling that he was talking about me. In all my memories of struggling with a speech block, the listeners I am trying to reach are my parents, and especially my father. I can remember the tears of frustration that filled my eyes when he told me, with the best of intentions, "Just slow down and relax." As for high expectations, it is a family joke that when I came home once from school to announce that the teacher had given me a ninety on a spelling test, my father asked, "Who got the other ten points?" And we were certainly as upwardly mobile as any other second-generation American Jewish household in the Bronx neighborhood where I grew up. But that is precisely the problem. My family had no monopoly on any of these traits. Many of my friends had similar relationships with their fathers. Why was I the only one who developed a stutter?

Not long ago, while I was having dinner at my parents' apartment, I asked them if they could remember exactly when I had started to stutter.

They looked surprised. As far as they could remember, they had never thought of me as a stutterer.

But hadn't they ever talked with someone at school—a teacher or a counselor or a speech therapist—about my speech problem?

Absolutely not. They had never been particularly concerned about the way I spoke—except for one time when I came home from summer camp with what sounded like a parody of a Brooklyn accent.

Well, then, did they remember trying to get me not to talk so fast?

Only when I was so excited or keyed up about something that I started stumbling over my words.

Did they remember when I first did that?

No.

Did they remember when I had stopped doing that?

"You were doing it just now," my father said. And, although I hadn't been aware of it a few moments before, I had to admit that he was right.

The nice thing about Johnson's diagnosogenic theory of stuttering is the implication that if just one generation of parents could stop worrying about the problem called stuttering, there would be no more stuttering to worry about. To keep the parents of young children from becoming part of the problem, Johnson offers this advice: Pay no attention whatsoever to your child's hesitancies and repetitions. At the same time, try to avoid any situation—excessive demands, overstimulation, fatigue—that seems to produce an unusual amount of "disfluency." When your child talks, be a good listener; respond to what he says, and let him know that speech can be "rewarding and fun."

Of course, none of this advice is much help to the adult who stutters, as Johnson knew only too well. If the child does not get over his stuttering by the end of adolescence, he may develop the mannerisms of the chronic stutterer—violent head jerks, arm-flailing, spasmodic breathing. Most of these mannerisms begin as attempts to break out of a speech block. Because of their novelty, they may actually help for a while. But in time they become part of the habit itself—the most visible and least attractive part. Once this stage is reached, more direct therapeutic measures are obviously called for; and, to judge from his autobiographical writings, Johnson tried them all. One of the strangest—to the ears of non-stutterers—was a technique developed at Iowa and known as "voluntary stuttering.'' This grew out of the theory that the best way to break a bad habit is to pretend to give in to it; by consciously trying to do what you previously tried to avoid doing, you somehow gain control over what began as an involuntary action. At first, Johnson had great success with this method. In between the periods when he was forcing himself to stutter, he was speaking more clearly than he had spoken at any time since early childhood. But when he stopped his periods of voluntary stuttering he lost all control and ended up virtually unable to say a word. It took "a week's moratorium on talking" to return him to his former level of semi-fluency.

Some of his colleagues—and fellow stutterers—had better luck with voluntary stuttering. One was a young man named Charles Van Riper, who took a Ph.D. in speech pathology at Iowa in 1936 and then left to set up a speech clinic and research center at what is now Western Michigan University. In adapting "Iowa therapy" to his own needs, Van Riper devised a method he called fluent stuttering. Essentially, he said to his students, "If you are going to stutter, at least learn to do it right." Since any stutterer knows that struggling with a block only makes it worse, Van Riper's students did not try to stop stuttering. Instead, they tried to stutter as smoothly as possible, without the spasmodic breathing, facial tics, or other muscular tensions that characterize the full-blown impediment.

Stuttering therapy as practiced in schools and university clinics in the United States today is based largely on Van Riper's version of Iowa therapy. Over the years, Van Riper has developed an elaborate battery of vocal tools that enable the stutterer to cancel a block or pull out of it before the continuity of the sentence is wrecked. A person trained in the Van Riper method may attack a Jonah word like "mother" by prolonging the first syllable into a long mooing sound. The result may not be exactly like normal speech, but it is better than trying to talk through sealed lips. For some reason, prolonging the vowel sound often gets the stutterer through the block and into the next word. And, because fluent stuttering requires the stutterer to keep making decisions, it forces him to pay attention to what Van Riper calls his "preparatory set"—the thoughts and feelings that run through him just before he comes to a Jonah word. This is the moment when, in Van Riper's words, "the brain that controls the mouth is flooded with static from the viscera." The job of the stutterer is to gain an objective view of what is happening and, ultimately, to replace the self-defeating preparatory set with a more functional model.

Members of the American Speech and Hearing Association—a fifty-year-old professional society which most speech therapists belong to—tend to be wary of any attempt to treat stuttering that departs radically from the Iowa approach. Having spent so many years exposing the charlatans who promise quick cures, the professional therapists especially distrust researchers who propose to cure the stuttering habit completely by some experimental method of conditioning or retraining.

Perhaps it was my own bias as an ex-stutterer, but the more I read about the legacy of Johnson (who died in 1965) and the work of Van Riper, the more uneasy I became. Here were two men, both severe stutterers, who had dominated the scientific study of their own impediment for nearly four decades. While no one could question their dedication, their objectivity was, to put it mildly, suspect. How could they keep an open mind about theories and therapies that had failed them? How could they help favoring the theories and therapies that had done them the most good?

Today, young researchers in the field will concede that very little work has been done on what modern medicine calls "differential diagnosis." A symptom like stuttering may be associated with more than one kind of disorder, just as an uncontrollable tremor of the hand can be a sign of nervous strain or a symptom of cerebral palsy. The treatment prescribed for a hand tremor will obviously depend on the diagnosis of a particular case. But until recently the usual assumption in speech therapy was that all people who stuttered (except those with obvious brain damage) did so for the same reason.

Even ex-stutterers may have difficulty dealing objectively with certain aspects of this maddening affliction. I find it hard to be objective about the fact that some Englishmen consider it a mark of good breeding to speak with a slight "stammer." Indeed, members of the upper classes who do not stammer often pretend that they do. There are stammerers in both houses of Parliament, and no one seems to know whose impediment is real and whose is affectation. To be sure, King George VI suffered greatly from his stammer, and both Winston Churchill and Aneurin Bevan worked hard to overcome their childhood speech impediments and win reputations for eloquence in the House of Commons. But some M.P.'s and Lords believe that a few judicious hesitations, repetitions, and prolongations can make a speaker seem more eloquent—apparently on the ground that a stammer holds the listener's attention and makes him grateful when something finally comes out.

To get the opinion of a non-stuttering expert on stuttering, I went to see Oliver Bloodstein, a well-known professor of speech at Brooklyn College, who is the author of *A Handbook on Stuttering*, an official publication of the National Easter Seal Society. In response to my first question, he estimated that more than 50 percent of his colleagues in stuttering research are stutterers themselves: "Many of them are amazed to find that someone who doesn't stutter can understand the problem." When I asked Bloodstein what a non-stutterer like him was doing in a field like this, he said that his choice of a career was something of an accident. As an undergraduate at the City College of New York during the Depression, he had majored in English (with a minor in speech) so that he could get a teaching job after graduation and support himself while he wrote poetry. But in 1941, when he graduated, there was a glut of English teachers in New York State, and one of his advisers suggested that he sign up instead for the graduate program in speech pathology at the University of

Iowa. Bloodstein had no particular interest in stuttering until he heard Wendell Johnson give a talk about the work at the Speech Clinic. "I was absolutely fascinated by the spectacle of this stuttering man talking about his research on stuttering. He was using a technique known as 'bouncing'—throwing caution to the winds, repetitions galore but no strain or tension. Considering the fact that he was stuttering, he was one of the most fluent people I had ever heard. I decided that I wanted to work with him."

Like Johnson, Bloodstein thinks that people stutter because they have been convinced that speech is difficult for them. But he tends to view the problem in an even wider context. Confidence is an essential ingredient of any act of physical coordination, whether it is walking, typing, playing the piano, or digging a ditch. Like all these, Bloodstein says, speaking a simple sentence is a "serially ordered act" that is usually carried out with a high degree of "automaticity." You cannot wait for each sound to emerge from your mouth before you consciously start to shape the next. Instead, you must treat an entire phrase as a unit, and work out a "motor plan" that determines in advance the sequence and timing of the necessary muscle movements. This is one of the skills a child must learn. But motor plans, like other well-laid plans, can fall apart under stress, leaving the speaker to cope with the disconnected fragments of language.

To make the point clear, Bloodstein drew a familiar analogy: Suppose someone places a wooden plank a foot wide and ten feet long on the floor of a room and asks you to walk from one end to the other. You do it easily, without thinking. Now suppose the plank is raised to the top of a brick wall that is a foot thick and twenty feet high. In purely physical terms, the task of walking from one end of the plank to the other has not been made any harder. But when you stand on one end and prepare to take your first step, you cannot help looking down and seeing the twenty-foot drop on both sides. And while you may tell yourself that your fear is unrealistic, you cannot help worrying about falling. And once you begin to worry, you start doing everything a little differently. Instead of maintaining a smooth, loose, automatic gait, you tighten your muscles, you lose your timing, and your movements become jerky, uneven, fragmented. Whereas your fear *was* unrealistic at first, now—as a direct result of your efforts to keep your balance—you find yourself in real danger of falling. And the harder you fight to regain control, the more helpless you become. In somewhat similar fashion, Bloodstein added, speed typists who go to work for unreasonably demanding bosses have been known to develop a "manual stutter"—they cannot type a letter without getting their fingers snarled on the keys.

For a young child who is still trying to master his speech skills, one factor that can cause a breakdown in verbal motor planning is too much social scrutiny. The child's fear of failure may not be realistic at first, but his desperate struggle not to fail, eventually leads to the muscular tension and fragmentation of speech units known as stuttering. At this point, anything that restores his confidence will improve his speech. So will anything that distracts him from the futile task of trying to exert conscious control over his speech organs. And so will anything that reduces the demands on his motor-planning skills during speech, such as singing the words to a familiar melody, reciting in unison with someone else, swinging dumbbells, pounding a drum—anything that establishes a steady, unmistakable beat and relieves the speaker of the responsibility for timing his own utterances. And yet "cures" based solely on distraction or rhythmical crutches cannot last, according to Bloodstein, because they do nothing to change the stutterer's self-defeating attitude.

A stutterer who is forced to say certain of his

Jonah words and sounds aloud can often prove to himself that he has trouble only when he anticipates trouble. Words beginning with "ph" offer a striking example. Some stutterers who are sure they cannot say the initial "f" in words like "folio" and "forward" will have no trouble at all reading aloud a word like "photo." Conversely, the sight of the word "photo" will choke up a stutterer who expects to have trouble with "p" words but never worries about words beginning with "f." The same kind of confusion occurs when stutterers who usually block on words beginning with the "s" sound are asked to read aloud a passage containing words like "cellar" and "sugar"; perversely, they breeze through the first word only to stumble over the second. Bloodstein told me about the time he asked a fifteen-year-old boy if there were any sounds that gave him particular trouble. The boy nodded, and said, "The d-d-d-d-d-double-u sound. See, I couldn't say it just now."

"The stutterers I work with often seem to be on the other side of a thin partition dividing them from normal speech," Bloodstein said. He believes that many young stutterers eventually stop stuttering without help because they outgrow their juvenile insecurities. For those who do not, supportive therapy in the Iowa style may be useful. "If there is any situation in which a stutterer is almost sure to stutter, it's when you ask him to repeat something," he said. "When you say to a stutterer 'What was that again?' you are implying that the responsibility for communication at that moment is his alone. Suddenly he's put on his mettle as a speaker, he feels that he has to make each word count, and he breaks down."

Everything that Bloodstein said struck me as sensible and plausible, but I still found the Iowa approach to "disfluency" faintly depressing. As a therapeutic tool, it seemed to concede too much to the enemy. And as theory it seemed too much of a patchwork—a psychological insight here, a contribution from sociology there, a little neurology, a little anthropology, a leavening of old-fashioned common sense. The whole appeared much less impressive than the individual parts—an appraisal that Van Riper himself has concurred with. "Most of the research on stuttering has been descriptive and, for therapy, rather sterile," he wrote a few years ago. "Some integrated attack on the problem is sorely needed." One of Van Riper's recent books on stuttering ends with a quotation from an article by Wendell Johnson that first appeared in 1944: "The chief justification for our present theories and methods is that we just don't know any better."

Potentially, the most exciting source of new

45

leads is brain research. But, while the study of the brain's role in language is fascinating in itself, the findings of the neuroscientists are still too sketchy to have many clinical applications. Most of what we know about the cerebral control of speech comes from the work of brain surgeons like the late Wilder Penfield, who performed more than five hundred operations at the Montreal Neurological Institute between 1934 and 1960. His patients were mostly people suffering from epileptic seizures that had been caused by local injury, infection, or lack of oxygen supply to the brain (anoxia). All these conditions can leave areas of damaged tissue on the surface or in the depths of the cerebral cortex—the convoluted layers of gray matter that cover the cerebral hemispheres. Removing the scarred areas can sometimes restore normal brain function. But it also involves some risk—excision of certain parts of the cortex can result in permanent loss of speech and other vital functions. To make sure that he was not trespassing on an indispensable area of the brain before he started to remove the tissue, Dr. Penfield developed a method of mapping the cortex before surgery. In a typical operation, the patient is given a local anesthetic in the scalp, and then the surface of the brain is exposed and different points on the

46

cortex are gently stimulated with the tip of an electrode. Each time the electrode touches the cortex, the reactions of the fully awake patient are carefully scrutinized. Since brain tissue itself does not feel anything, reactions occur only in those parts of the body which are controlled by the brain cells being stimulated. For example, in the voluntary-motor cortex—the area of the brain responsible for voluntary muscle movements—electrical stimulation invariably interrupts the patient's normal control over a limb or an organ. When one point in his cortex is stimulated, he finds himself lifting his right arm without having willed the action. If points in the sensory cortex are stimulated, the patient may report a tingling sensation in one toe or numbness in one finger. And in areas of the cortex that Penfield called "interpretive" the touch of an electrode can set off detailed psychic experiences. These are extraordinarily vivid snatches of memory, which the patient experiences almost as if he were sitting in a movie theater. One patient heard "the singing of a Christmas song in her church at home in Holland," Penfield reported in 1954. "She seemed to be there in the church and was moved again by the beauty of the occasion, just as she had been on that Christmas Eve some years before."

So strong are these visual and auditory impressions that the patient may feel as if he were "living through moments of past time," and yet, paradoxically, he remains aware of being in an operating room with an electrode on his brain. Another patient of Penfield's, who had recently come from his home in South Africa, cried out when his cortex was stimulated at one point, "Yes, Doctor! Yes, Doctor! Now I hear people laughing—my friends—in South Africa." When the stimulation ended, he said that "it had seemed to him that he was with his cousins at their home where he and the two young ladies were laughing together." During the stimulation, however, the patient had spoken to the doctor, not to the cousins. According to Penfield, this is the unvarying rule: "No patient has ever addressed himself to a person who was part of a past experience." In other words, stimulation of the interpretive areas of the cortex does not evoke speech directly; rather, it triggers "flashbacks" that, in turn, prompt the patient to comment on what he is seeing and hearing.

But there *are* two areas of the cortex that have been shown to be directly involved in speaking. These areas—known since the late nineteenth century as Broca's area and Wernicke's area—are on the side of the brain (usually the left) that is dominant for speech. People with tumors or lesions in these areas have trouble dealing with words as symbols—a condition known as aphasia. A person suffering from aphasia may be unable to make sense out of what is said to him, even though he can hear the separate sounds. Or he may be unable to frame a coherent reply to questions even though he can demonstrate by gestures that he knows what is expected of him. Aphasics will sometimes begin a sentence and then pause in confusion, unable to summon up the name of the most commonplace object, such as a chair or a spoon.

By using electrical stimulation, Penfield was able to map Broca's and Wernicke's areas with great precision in individual patients. In the course of his explorations, he discovered that the left side of the brain was dominant for speech in the great majority of his patients, whether they were right-handed or left-handed. Penfield also noted that under electrical stimulation the speech areas behaved quite differently from any of the other cortical areas he had mapped. No matter where the electrode touched down in Broca's or Wernicke's areas, there was never any "positive response to the stimulation," Penfield reported. "No movement is produced and no sensation. No positive psychical process [like a flashback] is set in motion. The stimulation does not summon words to the mind of the man nor does it cause him to speak. If he is lying quietly on the operating table, he has no means of knowing that the electrode has been applied to a speech area in his own dominant hemisphere. But if, at the moment of stimulation, the patient is speaking, he discovers, to his astonishment, that he is making mistakes. He may use some words but he cannot find others. Or, on the other hand, he may be speechless, though he tries to speak and perhaps snaps his fingers in exasperation. After withdrawal of the electrode, words may come with a rush, and he explains what he had been trying to say but could not."

One patient was shown a picture of a foot while an electrode touched his speech cortex. "Oh, I know what it is," he said. "That is what you put in your shoes." After the electrode was withdrawn, he said, "Foot!" Another time, the same patient seemed to be struggling to identify a picture of a butterfly. When the electrode was removed and he was able to talk again, he immediately gave the correct name, then remarked, "I couldn't get that word 'butterfly,' and then I tried to get the word 'moth.' "

Penfield also stimulated patients in the area of the motor cortex that controls articulation. When the electrode touched certain points, patients who were already talking began to vocalize—to give a sustained vowel cry. The effect was far more like a symptom of aphasia than like a stutter. In fact, Penfield's most important contribution to stuttering research was probably his finding that there is no single spot in the brain where the elements of speech are compactly stored. Try as he might, he could not evoke one intelligible word from any of his patients by electrical stimulation. At certain places in the brain, the touch of a single electrode could activate as well as suppress vigorous arm and leg movements, or turn on a vivid flashback in living color complete with sound track. But the summoning of even the simplest word apparently requires the coordination of several widely scattered control centers.

If nothing else, then, Penfield offered new proof that speech is an enormously complicated function—so complicated that we should not be surprised that it breaks down occasionally under one kind of stress or another. But the neurological evidence could not answer the two main questions: what are the specific conditions that cause a breakdown, and how can the damage be best repaired? In the last few years, a school of therapists who claim to have the answers has emerged from the relatively new field of behavioral therapy. If stuttering *is* learned in childhood, the behaviorist says, it can be unlearned later—not just in part but completely, and in a comparatively short time. One of the most forceful spokesmen for this viewpoint is Michael Webster, formerly the director of the Speech and Hearing Institute of New York and now director of the School of Human Communication Disorders at Dalhousie University, Halifax, Nova Scotia. Dr. Webster, who is fortyish and does not stutter, is clearly impatient with the failures of the past. He criticizes Van Riper's version of Iowa therapy for "not confronting the problem—they cover it up instead of taking it away," and he is openly skeptical about statistics purporting to show that large numbers of stutterers have been cured. "One of the most disconcerting things about attending professional meetings in this field is to go to the inevitable panel discussion featuring 'cured' stutterers and hear someone say, 'I was c-c-c-cured' by this or that method."

When I asked Webster what he thought about the high proportion of stuttering researchers who were stutterers, he shook his head. "We wouldn't think of going to a person with a bad lisp to learn not to lisp, but with stuttering it's been considered almost a guarantee of success," he said.

If the behavior therapists are hard on everyone else in the field, they are even harder on themselves. "When behavior therapy is unsuccessful," Webster says, "there are only three possible reasons: either the state of the art isn't far enough advanced, or the therapist is doing something wrong, or else he has misdiagnosed the case in the first place. In any event, the onus is on the therapist, not on the patient."

Some behavior therapists treat stuttering as a "speech phobia," not unlike such animal phobias as the morbid fear of snakes. The basic behavioral approach to the cure of phobias was pioneered in South Africa in the early fifties by Dr. Joseph Wolpe, who is now a professor of psychiatry at Temple University's School of Medicine. Wolpe "desensitized" his phobic patients the way an allergist desensitizes hayfever sufferers: by deliberately exposing them to carefully controlled doses of the thing they react to most violently. Wolpe's apparent success in curing phobias led two well-known speech pathologists, Eugene Brutten and Donald Shoemaker, to try to adapt his method to the treatment of stuttering. Just as some people break into a cold sweat every time they see a snake (or even a picture of a snake), other people begin to stutter whenever they have to pick up a ringing telephone and say hello. Brutten and Shoemaker argued that the mechanism in the two cases was the same. Once, probably in early childhood, something upset the patient so badly that he had a strong physical reaction—his skin turned clammy, he shook all over, his speech became uncoordinated. The moment passed, but the experience left its impression on the nervous system. Now whenever something happens that is reminiscent of the original episode, the phobic person cannot help having the same reaction. He has been conditioned in the classic Pavlovian sense. For example, a person with a snake phobia may actually have been bitten by a snake as a child, or he may simply have thought that a snake was going to bite him, or the image of a snake may have become associated in his mind with a trip to the country when his mother and father had a terrible quarrel and he was sure he was going to be abandoned. Similarly, a person with a speech phobia may have been severely punished for something he once said, or the act of speaking may somehow have become associated with a sense of loss, real or imagined.

The job of the behavior therapist is not to speculate on the cause of the phobia, however, but to remove the irrational fear. The whole point of the desensitization procedure is to set up conditions under which the patient can confront the feared stimulus without ever feeling afraid. Wolpe and other investigators have found that one of the best ways to combat a strong emotional reaction is to make sure that the patient is thoroughly relaxed to begin with; this often requires prior training in deep-muscle relaxation.

A person who is afraid of snakes may first be shown a cartoon of a cute, obviously harmless, Walt Disneyish reptile on a small projection screen at the far end of a room. If the conditions have been arranged correctly, the patient will be able to look at this picture without having a phobic reaction. (If he feels even the slightest wisp of "negative emotion," the cartoon will be immediately replaced with an even less threatening image, perhaps the letters "s-n-a-k-e" on a small flash card.) The next image should be just a little more realistic, and the next, and the next, until, by carefully graduated steps and without ever tripping the fear alarm in his mind, the patient is led to the point where he is able to stare at a live snake in a cage, or possibly even touch its scaly skin. He may not learn to love snakes, but the irrational chain of association linking snakes and terror has been severed, presumably forever.

Similarly, in Webster's laboratory, a stutterer

who has special difficulty using a telephone may be asked to set up and act out a hierarchy of increasingly uncomfortable situations. He may begin by whispering "Hello" into the mouthpiece of a toy phone. After going through all the motions on this toy, he may graduate to imaginary conversations on a real telephone whose cord has been cut, and then to actual conversations on a working phone. At each stage, he will begin with conversations that provoke the least anxiety (chatting with his wife or a good friend) and move gradually to the most upsetting situations (calling his boss to tell him he will be late for work, or asking a girl for a date, or calling a department store to complain about a mistake in a bill). When he reaches the point where using the telephone no longer bothers him, he may move on to other problem areas—meeting strangers at a party, giving instructions to a cabby, or whatever.

Systematic desensitization can be a slow, tedious process. Since the idea is always to move from success to success, the steps in each hierarchy must be small enough to insure that the patient never has reason to doubt his ability to handle the next challenge. In an effort to speed up the process without overburdening the patient, many therapists are now combining desensitization with methods devised to coax fluent speech out of even the most severely blocked stutterers. For example, Dr. John Paul Brady, chairman of the psychiatry department at the University of Pennsylvania, has developed a battery-operated electronic metronome that fits behind the ear as unobtrusively as a hearing aid. The metronome sounds a pleasant tone in the stutterer's ear at so many beats a minute. By twisting a control on the small, self-contained unit, the stutterer can vary the rate from forty beats a minute on up to 150 beats a minute. The stutterer uses this tone—which only he can hear—to time his utterances, fitting one syllable to each beat. In normal conversation, a non-stutterer articulates between 120 and 200 words a minute. If a stutterer tried to talk that fast, he would almost certainly become blocked. But virtually every stutterer can talk without blocking if he lets the metronome cue each syllable for him, and if he sets the pace slow enough to begin with. Once he gains confidence at a particular pace—sixty beats a minute, perhaps—he gradually increases it until he is able to talk fluently at a normal rate in all situations that once gave him trouble. He is then encouraged to give up the metronome—not all at once but gradually, first by reducing the volume until he can barely hear the tone, then by leaving the device off at times when he anticipates no unusual challenges. Most patients find that after several months they can get through an entire day without mechanical cues—presumably because they have learned to time their speech internally the way other people do. But since the metronome device is small and comparatively inexpensive, the stutterer can keep it at hand in case he ever feels the need for it; just knowing that it is available may help prevent the relapses that undermine so many other apparent cures for stuttering.

There is another school of stuttering therapists who combine the systematic use of desensitization and related training regimes with insights borrowed from the science of cybernetics. Their basic assumption is that speech can best be understood as the output of a servomechanism—that is, a device with built-in feedback loops which continuously monitors its own performance and modifies its activity accordingly. The most obvious feedback loop for speech control is hearing. If I hear myself mispronounce a word or garble a concept, I can stop and repeat the word or try to reformulate the concept. At the same time, I am also monitoring my speech through other sensory channels—the vibrations in my facial bones, the way the muscles in my throat, mouth, and face feel when I articulate a certain sound, the response I read on the face of the person I am talking to. Servomechanisms can reach and sustain a high level of performance as long as all their components are working properly. But anyone who has ever heard the screech of an improperly tuned loudspeaker system knows how much trouble even a minor flaw in a feedback loop can cause.

The effect of faulty feedback on speech control was first demonstrated in 1949 by an acoustical engineer named Bernard S. Lee. The discovery was accidental, and the experience was traumatic, according to Lee, who is now a member of the faculty at the Rutgers Medical School and devotes all his time to research on stuttering. Lee was working for the Army Signal Corps in 1949, and one of his duties was to check new equipment that came into the laboratory, at Fort Monmouth, New Jersey. He had just received a new magnetic tape recorder that had two separate heads, one for recording and one for playback, and two earphone jacks, one for monitoring input during recording and one for listening to the playback. By mistake, Lee plugged his earphones into the playback jack while he was talking into the microphone. Since the tape reached the playback head a fraction of a second after it passed through the recording head, he heard his own voice coming back to him with a fraction-of-a-second delay. The tight-fitting earphones blocked out all normal auditory feedback, so when he said, "Testing, one, two, three," he could hear himself only on the tape. But because of the delay, this feedback had a surreal quality. For example, he heard nothing at all until he had finished saying "Testing, one . . ." Then he heard his voice saying the word "testing" just as he started to say "two," and heard himself saying "one" just as he started to say "three." At first, he had no idea of what was happening. When he tried to keep talking, he felt his control slipping. He recalls, "My voice started quavering. I started slurring my words, I was blocking, repeating things, and I had a rotten feeling inside. At first, I thought it was mike fright." It took Lee half an hour to calm down after the experience. Then he went back to the machine, found the earphones plugged into the wrong jack, and realized that he had been a victim of faulty feedback. In a paper he published the following year in the *Journal of the Acoustical Society of America*, he described his reaction as an "artificial stutter."

Further investigation revealed that not everyone stuttered under the influence of what soon became known as "delayed auditory feedback," or simply D.A.F. In fact, some severe stutterers began to speak more fluently when they put the earphones on—a finding that led one researcher to design an entire therapeutic program around the use of D.A.F. Only one general rule applied to the experience: it was impossible to maintain a normal rate of speech under D.A.F. People who did not stutter tended to slow down drastically, as if they were imitating a 45-r.p.m. record played at 33-r.p.m. I tried it myself in Lee's laboratory at Rutgers and found that the slowing down was quite involuntary. As soon as my voice started coming to me out of synch with what I knew I was saying, I became eerily aware of my lips and facial muscles: I could feel my lips forming each "w" and "m" sound; I could feel my tongue slip into place for each "t" and "b" sound; and so on. Perhaps because I was concentrating so hard on this tactile feedback instead of on the D.A.F. signals, I did not stutter.

Oddly, Lee himself makes no use of delayed auditory feedback in the new stuttering therapy that he has been developing, in collaboration with a psychiatrist, Dr. W. Edward McGough, and a speech pathologist, Maryann Peins. But Lee does use tape recorders. In fact, his entire therapeutic program is recorded on a series of twelve cassettes, which can be played on any cassette machine. The stutterer is supposed to take each cassette home and carry on a dialogue with the recorded voice of the therapist while taping his own responses on a cassette in a second machine. After daily practice for two weeks, the stutterer returns the cassette to the therapist, discusses any special problems he may have had, and takes home the next lesson in the series.

It all sounds very McLuhanesque and machine-oriented. But the taped lessons themselves contain nothing that would not be perfectly comprehensible to Alexander Melville Bell—or, for that matter, to Demosthenes. There are word drills, and exercises for certain sounds, and simulated conversations, and little scenarios for extemporaneous speaking. But first the stutterer is taught to speak in a new way—a smooth, flowing style of continuous vocalization that Lee has termed "legato speech," but that earlier generations of speech therapists knew as "slurred" or "drawled" speech. As Lee teaches it, the whole trick is to get your vocal cords vibrating in a low, steady drone before you form your first word and then to keep up the drone as long as you keep speaking. The opposite of legato speech is staccato speech—the machine-gun-like delivery of short bursts of vocalization. The average speaker may not have any trouble speaking this way; the stutterer apparently does, for reasons still unknown. (Lee leans toward the view that stuttering is caused by some "instrumental defect" in the speech feedback system.) Lee does not claim that this method will work for everyone who stutters. But cassette therapy is certainly more economical than conventional face-to-face therapy, and a controlled study has shown that it works at least as well for many stutterers. Some even prefer it, because they have less trouble talking back to a faceless tape recorder than to a therapist.

Unlike some of the gimmicks that stutterers rely on to "loosen their tongues"—interjections like "um" and "ah" and "let me see"—legato speech draws no attention to itself. Radio announcers and ministers use it all the time, as do professional singers; the low steady drone between words is heard only as a pleasing fullness of tone. Lee, who is well aware of the historical parallels, is not sure why legato speech is so effective in helping stutterers build a beachhead of fluent speech. Nonstop vocalization may be easier for stutterers because it gives them one less variable to worry about; they just turn their voice on and leave it on. And there is no question that it forces them to speak more slowly—which Lee thinks may be the most important benefit of all.

I asked him why he thought so, and he said that experiments have repeatedly shown that talking faster always makes a bad stutter worse. The evidence from statistical surveys seems to bear this out. When a large group of ex-stutterers were asked what they attributed their recovery to, many of them said that they had simply learned to speak more slowly.

I told Lee that what he was saying reminded me of the advice that my parents gave me all through childhood; it may have been good advice, but I had not been prepared to accept it—at least, not when it came from my parents.

Lee asked what I had done to stop stuttering. I said that I couldn't remember doing anything in particular.

"Are you aware that you're speaking in a natural legato style?" he asked.

I said that I had not even been aware of the term until I came across it a few weeks before in one of his papers. But as I answered him I was listening to my voice, and in between the words I could hear the steady drone of vocalization, almost like the hum of an electronic amplifier between sets at a rock concert.

It is possible that I somehow stumbled on this trick while I was growing up, and unconsciously adopted it. But it doesn't seem possible that such a little change could have cut the knot that bound my speech. More likely, I learned to speak in legato style at the same time that I was gaining confidence in myself in other ways, and progress in one area reinforced progress in the others.

Another form of stuttering therapy that emphasizes the role of the vocal cords is the "airflow technique" of Martin F. Schwartz, research associate professor at New York University Medical Center. Schwartz believes that all stuttering is caused by trying to speak while the vocal cords are clamped shut in what he calls a laryngospasm. To make sure the cords are open and relaxed, he teaches his patients to sigh audibly just before speaking. Schwartz claims that when this is done properly—without trying to *push* the air out—the vocal cords cannot go into a spasm and a person cannot stutter. The trick, of course, is to get the patient into the habit of sighing before speaking so that he does not forget it even under great stress. According to Schwartz, the patient must practice airflow technique one hour a day for a whole year; during this time, various kinds of supportive therapy may be necessary to keep the patient on the right track and help him deal with stress-inducing situations.

Like Lee's legato speech, the core of Schwartz's technique—the passive sigh—was familiar to therapists in the nineteenth century, some of whom prescribed "breathy" speech to get the flow of words started. There is no question that such "starter" devices can be effective in the proper context; and a number of speech therapists and former patients have testified to the effectiveness of Schwartz's therapeutic package. There is also no question that Schwartz has been unrestrained, critics might say irresponsible, in espousing his method as "a revolutionary new treatment with an 89 percent success rate for both children and adult stutterers." These words are writ large on the front cover of his book, called *Stuttering Solved*, in which his summary of the history of stuttering research might lead the reader to conclude that no one had done any worthwhile work until Schwartz arrived on the scene. He has also appeared on TV talk shows to make the same pitch. All this hyperbole may turn out to be justified; only time—and unbiased follow-up studies—will tell. But, for the moment, his behavior has drawn the fire of his colleagues, who believe that a genuine contribution to medical science does not have to be promoted in the accents of Madison Avenue.

I suspect that neither I nor anyone else will ever be able to say exactly why I started to stutter or why I stopped. But with the spread of the Gospel According to Johnson—"Suffer little children to learn to talk at their own pace"—and with the number of therapeutic tools now available, and with the new emphasis on differential diagnosis to apply those tools more efficiently, it seems possible that there will be fewer and fewer people worrying about the problem called stuttering. Or writing letters such as one received by an internationally known speech therapist in New York a while ago. The writer was a twenty-four-year-old Turk, self-taught in several languages, including English, who wanted to know if there was anyone in America who could cure his stutter. "I love people, anything, everybody in the world but it is a bad judgment on me that I can't get around them," the letter said. "The fact is that I have to do something about it. . . . Otherwise a bullet through the head will do the thing. . . . I have many talents. But what's the use of knowing 2 or

3 languages unless you have the chance of any practice. . . . . Please help me out of this hell's torment. I can't stand it any more. I don't want to be an outcast in society."